NATURAL
LIVER THERAPY

Herbs and Other Natural Remedies for a Healthy Liver

by Christopher Hobbs

Botanica Press, Capitola, CA

**Other books in the "Herbs and Health" series
by Christopher Hobbs:**

Echinacea! The Immune Herb

Ginkgo, Elixir of Youth

Milk Thistle: The Liver Herb

Vitex: The Women's Herb

Valerian, The Relaxing Herb

Usnea, The Herbal Antibiotic

Medicinal Mushrooms

Handbook For Herbal Healing

Copyright September, 1986
2nd revision March, 1988
3rd revision September, 1993
4th printing April, 1995

by Christopher Hobbs

Michael Miovic, Editor
Beth Baugh, Project Editor
Plant illustrations copyright Donna Cehrs, Sept. 1992
Anatomy illustration by Francine Martin
Liver illustration copyright Marni Fylling, Sept. 1993

Botanica Press
Box 742
Capitola, CA 95010

TABLE OF CONTENTS

Author's Disclaimer

The information given in this book is for educational purposes and is not meant as a prescription for any specific ailment. If you have a serious illness, the author recommends seeking the services of a qualified, licensed health professional. Unless a statement is specifically referenced, it could be the author's opinion, based on extensive study and personal experience.

Our Commitment

We at Botanica Press are dedicated in our personal and professional lives to environmental awareness. We are strongly committed to recycling, and we gladly contribute a portion of our profits to the Nature Conservancy and other conservation groups. This book is printed on recycled paper with a minimum of 10% post-consumer waste, and the entire text is printed using soy-based ink.

Recycle
Conserve

This book is printed on Simpson 60lb recycled paper.

INTRODUCTION

The liver is a remarkable organ and is largely unappreciated for the many vital functions it performs. It has been said that it is not called the live-r for nothing: it keeps us living. The importance of keeping the liver open, healthy, and functioning smoothly is understood by doctors and herbalists alike. The liver is the major organ of digestion and assimilation, helping to provide the nutrients that maintain health and repair diseased or damaged tissue. It also provides a vital function in helping to eliminate toxic wastes from the body.

Unfortunately, however, liver disease is currently the fourth most common cause of death in this country, after cancer, heart disease, and strokes. This tragic situation could be prevented with proper dietary habits and natural liver therapy. The aim of this booklet is to present practical, up-to-date information about effective ways to regain and maintain optimal liver health. Specifically, we will look at:

- How the liver works, both in scientific terms and according to traditional Chinese medicine

- How fat, oils, and common foods affect the liver

- Herbal remedies for a variety of liver disorders

- Liver flushes and other natural methods for maintaining a healthy liver.

This book has a two-part format. The first part is the "theory" part. Here we'll examine what the liver does and how it does it. I have made every effort to make the scientific details understandable to the lay reader. The second part of the book—which may be of more immediate interest to many people—is the hands-on, "practical" part. Here I present useful information about what you can actually do to maintain liver health. I also describe diagnostic signs and symptoms, dietary recommendations, and herbal formulas for ten different liver-related disorders. I sincerely hope this information will benefit you and your loved ones. However, one word of caution—though I encourage independent experimentation, I also recommend that you seek the advice of a qualified natural health practitioner for difficult or long-standing liver problems. In any case, good luck on your healing journey!

HOW THE LIVER WORKS

THE LIVER'S JOB AND JOB STRESS

The liver's job, in a nutshell, is to make sure that the body absorbs everything it needs and dumps everything it doesn't. If one were to write a sort of job description for the liver, its list of major duties would look like this:

- Metabolizes proteins, fats, and carbohydrates, thus providing energy and nutrients

- Stores vitamins, minerals, and sugars

- Filters the blood and helps remove harmful chemicals and bacteria

- Creates bile, which breaks down fats

- Helps assimilate and store fat-soluble vitamins (A, E, D, K)

- Stores extra blood, which can be quickly released when needed

- Creates serum proteins, which maintain fluid balance and act as carriers

- Helps maintain electrolyte and water balance

- Creates immune substances, such as gamma globulin

- Breaks down and eliminates excess hormones

As you can see, that's a lot of work for a single organ to do even under the best of conditions. Unfortunately, however, the modern lifestyle burdens the liver with many stresses, making its job even more difficult.

After the insult of oily, processed foods, one of the major stress-factors the liver must contend with today is human-made chemicals, such as lead from gasoline, countless food additives, preservatives, pesticides, herbicides, and many other new compounds. It is estimated that chemical companies, in their search for marketable compounds, produce hundreds of new chemicals every year. Since these compounds are completely new to the environment, it may be thousands of years before our bodies evolve and adapt to them.

Other common liver stress-factors are alcohol and recreational drugs which are prevalent in the United States. Current figures estimate 15.1 million alcoholics and 22 million drug abusers in this country (U.S. Congress Report, Jan. 1987; National Clearing House on Drug Addiction, 1991). Furthermore, since drugs administered for therapeutic purposes also affect the liver, 5% of hospital patients in the United States (1.9 million people) develop significant adverse reactions to drugs administered by doctors. In fact, 2-4% of all hospital admissions (760,000 to 1.5 million people) are for doctor-prescribed drug reactions.

A final stress our livers must contend with is excess hormones, such as adrenalin, which are constantly being created in our bodies in response to our fast-paced modern lifestyle. Under some circumstances, hormones can be stored by the liver for up to a year, adding fuel to emotional imbalances such as depression and anger, as well as to stress-related imbalances such as immune-system depression.

THE LIVER AND DETOXIFICATION

So how exactly does the liver detoxify all the potentially harmful substances that are either put into or created in the body? In order to understand this, we must understand some basic chemistry. Many of the foreign and toxic chemicals that enter the body (either by descending through the food chain into the food we eat, or by direct intake of contaminants) are called lipid-soluble. This means they dissolve only in fatty or oily solutions, not in water. Lipid-soluble compounds have a special affinity for fat tissues and many other cells of the body which have lipid-soluble membranes, such as liver cells. These cells and tissues can store toxins for months, even years, releasing them during times of low food intake, exercise, or stress. As toxins are released, one may experience unpleasant symptoms such as tiredness, dizziness, nausea, racing pulse, etc.

It is the liver's job to transform lipid-soluble chemicals into water-soluble compounds so that they can be released via the kidneys and bowels. This transformation is carried out by a complex system of enzymes that are made in the hepatocytes, or liver cells.

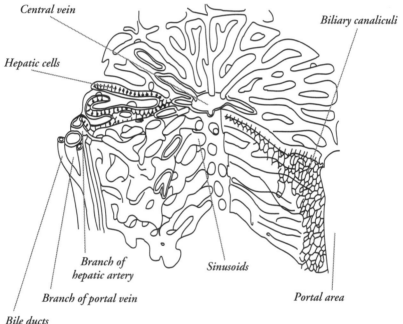

Besides having a complex system of enzymes to remove toxic compounds from the blood, the liver also has filtering channels, called sinusoids, that are lined with special cells which engulf and break down foreign debris, bacteria, and toxic chemicals (this process is called phagocytosis). However, when the liver is burdened with high levels of toxic chemicals or pathogenic organisms (such as *Candida albicans*, a major factor in yeast infections), not all of these substances can be processed and eliminated. In fact, many will be stored in the liver, eventually causing irreparable damage.

As you can see, it makes good sense that, in natural healing, the liver is considered to be an important organ in maintaining clean blood, because it actually does act as a sort of blood filter. Many herbalists call certain herbs good "blood purifiers." Does this mean these herbs literally scrub the blood clean? Not really. What actually happens is that the herbs stimulate increased blood flow through the liver, removing debris, old cells, toxins, etc. At the same time, they protect and stimulate the liver cells, thus encouraging the production of enzymes and helping to maintain a proper biochemical environment.

Of course, the liver is not the only organ involved in detoxification. Blood purification also depends upon the proper functioning of all the eliminative organs in the body. The skin, for instance, eliminates large quantities of toxins through sweating. That's why sweating therapy and increased fluid intake can often take a load off the liver. Finally, blood purifiers activate the immune system, such as the macrophages ("big eaters") which also help remove undesirable elements from the blood.

AN AMAZING CHEMICAL FACTORY

The liver is really an amazing chemical factory, and some of its workings deserve further discussion.

VITAMINS

Vitamins, minerals, and enzymes are vital to cellular health. They are the "messengers" and "currency" that help make things happen—from the creation of new cells, to the making of sexual hormones, to the release of energy. Significantly, the liver stores vitamins and minerals for times when they would otherwise be lacking. It can store enough vitamin A to supply an adult's needs for up to four years and enough vitamin D and vitamin B-12 to last for four months!

BILE

The liver also creates bile which helps break down fats by emulsifying them. Emulsification is a process that transforms large fat globules into tiny ones which are more water-soluble and assimilable (incidentally, this is the same process by which detergent cleans grimy, oily clothes). To help the liver with this process, a moderate walk after a meal rich in fat is desirable. This encourages the fat to move through the body and facilitates its processing.

Excessive amounts of fat and protein in the diet are difficult for the liver to break down because they make the liver work harder to produce bile and other digestive enzymes. In addition, ammonia produced by the metabolic breakdown of protein can irritate or even be toxic to the liver. Thus, when the liver is not functioning properly, or if it is diseased, it is important to eat fewer foods that contain fat and protein, such as meat and dairy products. It is also good to eat more easily assimilated complex carbohydrates, such as rice or millet, because these decrease the amount of bile needed and thus take a great load off the liver. This will also help to build up and better utilize glycogen (the storage form of glucose) in the hepatocytes, which means the liver will have more energy to rebuild itself and establish proper harmony.

One major cause of impaired bile flow is gallstones. Current medical literature states that at least 20 million people in the United States have gallstones. Bile stagnation can also result from actual cellular damage to the liver due to the negative effects of alcohol; hyperthyroidism or thyroxine supplementation; exposure to toxic drugs or other synthetic chemicals; and the use of birth control pills. When the bile is stagnant, the skin becomes sallow, yellow, or blemished. Also, important vitamins are not assimilated properly, which can impair blood clotting, vision, and the body's antioxidant system. Further damage to the body may occur when toxic compounds that are usually cycled through the bile and eliminated are held in the liver instead.

Many ancient systems of healing recognized the fact that bile is a vital bodily fluid. Herbs are commonly taken throughout the world to restore proper bile flow, for when the bile is stagnant, sadness and disharmony can result. The word "melancholy," for instance, comes from the Greek melanos (black) and chole (bile)—or literally, "black bile." This condition has been called "sluggish liver" in Western medicine and "liver stagnation" in Traditional Chinese Medicine (TCM).

ENZYMES

An enzyme is a complex protein that speeds up a chemical reaction in the body. Many (indeed most) of the chemical reactions that are going on inside us every second would not happen naturally unless the various reactants were heated up to high temperatures. That is because the reactions of life generally require a great deal of energy in order to proceed. However, enzymes allow these critical reactions to occur at body-temperature. Each enzyme (there are thousands of different kinds!) has its own, unique shape that allows it to "fit" with only certain molecules, like pieces of a jigsaw puzzle. When an enzyme attaches to its matching molecule, it can help break it into smaller pieces, or it can "glue" many smaller molecules together into a larger one. Thus enzymes speed up the chemical reactions involved in both the building up and breaking down (digestion) of substances in the body.

That is a working definition of what enzymes are. As we have already seen, during the detoxification process the liver makes use of various enzymes. Actually, these are not individual enzymes but whole enzyme systems, collectively named the Microsomal Enzyme System (MES). The MES is part of our evolutionary legacy. Its job is to process many different kinds of chemicals, as already explained. Most likely, the liver developed these enzyme systems to deactivate and facilitate the elimination of naturally-occurring, endogenous (i.e., produced within the body) chemicals such as bilirubin, serotonin, and the hormones estradiol and testosterone. The MES probably also evolved to help detoxify and eliminate many natural toxins present in the wild and in slightly spoiled foods, which were common before the advent of refrigeration.

Although the MES is necessary for survival, it is something of a two-edged sword. On the one hand, it can transform fat-soluble toxic chemicals, such as DDT, into more water-soluble ones that are easily eliminated via the bowels and urine. But on the other hand, ironically, the MES can also transform certain non-toxic compounds into toxic or even carcinogenic ones. For example, toxic alkaloids found in the medicinal plant comfrey are probably harmless until they travel through the liver and are transformed into highly potent compounds that can lead to liver damage (hence both researchers and herbalists now recommend caution in the use of comfrey products, especially during pregnancy).

HOW THE LIVER WORKS

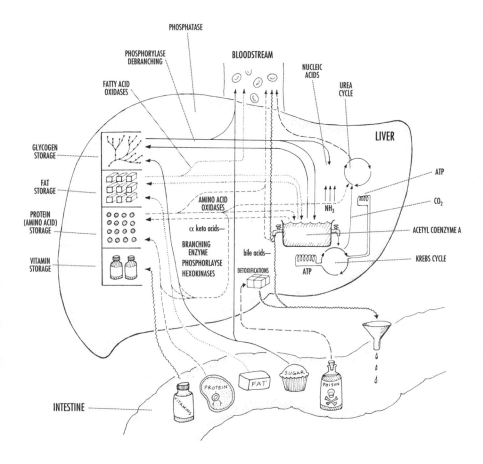

Now the different kinds of enzyme systems in the MES have been classified into two types: Phase I and Phase II systems. Phase I systems alter chemical groups on the foreign substance, rendering it more water-soluble and hence disposable. Phase II systems, in contrast, generally help to conjugate (or bind) a compound with sulfur-containing groups, presumably to make them less toxic, or as in the case of endogenous hormones, to deactivate them.

An example of a Phase I enzyme system is the Mixed-Function Oxidases (MFO) system, part of which is the Cytochrome P-450 system. Cytochrome P-450 plays a central role in detoxifying numerous potentially hazardous compounds. It also assists the synthesis of steroid hormones and, with vitamin C, works in an important step of bile synthesis. Unfortunately for the liver, however, certain toxic chemicals disrupt the P-450 system. These include common herbicides and pesticides, as well as breakdown products from them that can linger in the environment for many years (for instance DDE, a breakdown product from DDT, is still abundant in the environment many years after DDT was banned). These can be stored in fat tissues and slowly released into the bloodstream, eventually finding their way to the liver. Because the production of synthetic pesticides exceeds 1.4 billion pounds a year in this country, it is likely that there are enough toxic substances in the environment to adversely affect our livers and lives.

Phase II systems, for their part, include both UDP-glucuronyl transferase (GT), and glutathione-S-transferase (GSH-T). Glutathione (GSH-T) is one of the most important endogenous antioxidants and cellular protectors in the body. It can be depleted by large amounts of drugs or toxic chemicals passing through the liver, as well as by fasting or starvation. GSH-T is also subject to circadian rhythms, which means that its levels increase and decrease according to the body's 24-hour biological cycles. Thus there is 30% less GSH-T in the body in the late afternoon than late at night.

So what does all this mean for our health? Well, while natural amounts of substances such as GT and GSH-T are vital to optimal liver functioning, excessive amounts may be harmful. High GSH-T levels in the liver can cause non-toxic chemicals to be transformed into more toxic ones that damage the liver (Salbe and Bjeldanes, 1985). Thus, there must be just enough GHS-T available for important enzymatic reactions, but not so much as to cause excessive transformations. Or, in other words, health depends upon biochemical tone. Tone means that there is just enough of a particular substance, action, or force to maintain a state of dynamic equilibrium in the body, and consequently the ability to function. The Chinese call this the balance of Yin and Yang, but many Westerners prefer the concept of tone. Some simple but effective ways to maintain proper tone in the GSH-T and the liver's other enzyme systems include exercise, positive attitude, visualization, polarity therapy, and various other common methods for bringing about greater health. Also, we can use herbs and diet, which we shall soon address in depth.

THE LIVER AND EMOTIONAL BALANCE

In the preceding pages we have discussed a lot of technical and scientific concepts. How do these relate to the everyday lives of thinking, feeling human beings? Well, most importantly, any emotions one feels have a basis in biochemistry. When you feel angry, for instance, a complex mixture of hormones and other chemicals speed to various parts of your body, readying you for action. Likewise fear, jealousy, joy, sorrow, and all our other emotions have a corresponding chemical reality which can create profound changes in our bodies. And depending on the strength and duration of emotions, these changes can more or less determine one's character and outlook on life.

Thus, an important function of the liver, which is just now beginning to be understood, is its role in transforming and removing excess hormones from the blood. When the liver is diseased or is functioning poorly, its ability to do this is impaired. Then emotional states that should come and go easily stay around far longer than necessary. If one's environment is full of negative or excessive emotions, this burdens the liver.

Take anger, for instance. Traditional Chinese Medicine (TCM) holds that anger is associated with the liver and gallbladder (in a Western view we would say that the bile in the gallbladder can store the excess hormones not eliminated by a poorly functioning liver). Similarly, Ayurvedic medicine associates anger with the fire principle and the liver. Thus in either case someone who is chronically angry would be said to have an unhealthy liver or gallbladder. The prescribed treatment would be gentle opening, cleansing, and perhaps cooling of the bile and liver, using herbs and liver flushes (we will discuss all of these in detail later).

THE LIVER AND PMS

Having understood this much about the liver and emotions, it should be easy to grasp their connection with premenstrual syndrome (PMS). Currently, PMS is being linked to excess estrogen, a steroid hormone. Again, it is the liver's job to clear away any excess estrogen circulating through the body. However, if the body produces too much estrogen, the liver may not be able to keep up with its job, resulting in PMS symptoms, such as depression, cramps, headaches, fatigue, or even more serious problems. For instance, excess estrogen has been reported to increase the risk of gallbladder disease, production of clots and inflammation in the blood vessels, high blood pressure, hyperglycemia, and breast, uterine, liver, and vaginal cancer (*Physician's Desk Reference*, 1933). Current research is emphasizing that circulating estrogen levels in both men and women may be increased by environmental and dietary factors such as electromagnetic radiation (from appliances, power lines, etc.), herbicides and pesticides (Raloff, 1993), and alcohol consumption.

Fortunately, natural liver therapy can help with all types of hormonal imbalances, including PMS. For women who do not produce enough estrogen and consequently receive prescribed estrogen therapy (as for osteoporosis and symptoms associated with menopause), it is especially important to support the liver with natural liver therapy during times when estrogen is taken. As for those who suffer from estrogen excess leading to emotional swings, food cravings, and other undesirable symptoms, natural plant remedies can block the binding sites estrogen normally uses to activate or modify cellular processes in estrogen-sensitive tissue. In this way, natural plant remedies can prevent estrogen from over-extending the scope and amount of its beneficial activities (Farnsworth, 1980).

Besides estrogen, testosterone, too, is metabolized by the liver. Testosterone normally exists in both the male and female body and is known to affect levels of aggressiveness and sexual energy. Hence if the liver cannot properly eliminate excess testosterone, over-aggressiveness, extreme mood swings, and abnormal levels of sexual energy may result, as well as dysfunction of the reproductive cycle.

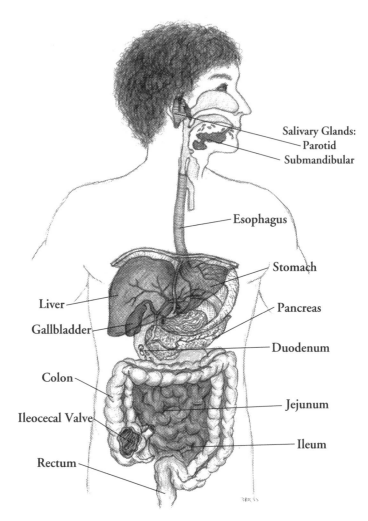

The Human Digestive Tract

THE CHINESE LIVER SYSTEM

So far we have discussed the liver as it is known to Western science. The concept of the liver in Traditional Chinese Medicine (TCM) is somewhat different and merits closer study.

The ancient healing system of TCM recognizes five bodily systems, each of which is associated with one of the five primary elements in nature. Also, each of the principal internal organs is thought to be connected to an external part of the body which it affects, to an external anatomical part where the condition of the internal organ is reflected and to an emotion and climatic condition. Table 1 summarizes these basic relationships.

TABLE 1.

THE FUNDAMENTAL RELATIONSHIPS OF TCM

ORGAN SYSTEM	ELEMENT	DIAGN. PART	AFFECTED PARTS	CLIMATE	TASTE	EMOTIONS
stomach/spleen	earth	mouth	flesh, lips	moisture	sweet	self-pity
lungs/colon	metal	nasal cavities	skin/body hair	dryness	acrid	grief, despair
kidney/bladder	water	ears, hair head	bones,	coldness	salty	fear, anxiety
liver/gallbladder	wood	eyes	tendons, nails, ligaments	wind	sour	anger
heart/ pericardium/ small intestine	fire	tongue	vascular system complexion	heat	bitter	excitement, fright

According to TCM, the liver's main job is to regulate the flow of chi (chi means, approximately, "life energy"). Chi is responsible for all activity of the body, the blood, the chi itself, and for proper functioning of the organs. The liver moves the blood and chi smoothly in all directions throughout the body and harmonizes the functioning of the organs. Naturally, then, the liver is particularly sensitive to anything that disrupts what the Chinese so aptly call its "free and easy wanderer" movement and influence within the body. Excessive or negative emotions, especially, will disrupt this free-flowing ambiance, leading to conditions of deficiency, coldness, or stagnation. The net result of any such blockage of energy in the liver is a buildup of toxins, which can cause cellular damage and poor functioning of the Microsomal Enzyme System (MES) we discussed earlier. This in turn may lead to further damage from free radicals and peroxidized lipids, which we shall address later.

As well as being susceptible to blockage or chi stagnation, the liver is also susceptible to over-stimulation. In the latter condition, the liver receives too much blood and goes into a sort of metabolic overdrive called "blazing fire" in TCM. This state can be caused by alcohol, drugs, and an excess of certain spices, such as black pepper. Blazing fire can remain localized in the liver and cause overheating, which in Western terms may lead to enzyme dysfunction and damage to the hepatocytes. Or the heat can rise up to the head, inducing headaches, facial flushing, thirst, dizziness, and ringing in the ears.

The liver has other important functions in TCM in addition to regulating the flow of chi in the body. First of all, it regulates digestive activity. When the liver fails in this task due to loss of biochemical harmony, its action can "invade," or negatively affect, the stomach, thus precipitating digestive problems such as abdominal pain, nausea, burping, and diarrhea.

Secondly, in TCM just as in Western medicine, the liver also controls the bile. If the bile does not flow smoothly, jaundice, loss of appetite, and a bitter taste in the mouth will result. Fats will not be well tolerated or assimilated, and the fat-soluble vitamins A, E, D, and K will not be utilized well—which could lead to immune depression.

Thirdly, the liver harmonizes the emotions. According to some TCM texts, it has a "sprinkling" movement that is responsible for maintaining a relaxed and flowing inner environment and an even-tempered disposition. This works in a cyclic way: a healthy liver helps maintain an even temperament, and vice versa. However, if the cycle turns downward, a turbulent emotional climate can damage the liver, and the injured liver will further aggravate the emotional chaos.

A fourth important function of the liver, understood by TCM and Western medicine alike, is to store extra blood for use in times of need, as during physical activity. However, according to TCM, imbalances occur if the liver either does not have enough extra blood stored (resulting in dryness in the eyes), or if it loses its ability to store blood properly (resulting in excessive menstrual flow).

Lastly, it is important to note that TCM texts state that the liver also "rules" the tendons and is manifested in the nails. This can provide helpful diagnostic information. For example, if the tendons are stiff, hard, and painful, or if the nails are pale and brittle, then it could mean that the liver is failing to nourish them properly.

Remember that in TCM all these aspects of liver functioning are interrelated, so that in reality no one aspect can be separated from the others. We only look at them separately because this helps us to draw conclusions about functional disharmony and successful treatment.

NATURAL LIVER THERAPY

GENERAL DIETARY GUIDELINES

Now that we have a fairly good idea of how the liver does its work, let's take a look at what a person can do to maintain optimum liver health. First we'll discuss dietary factors and practices that everyone should consider. Even if you aren't suffering from any obvious liver disorder at the moment, good eating habits can save you from developing problems later. After examining diet, we'll then address herbal therapies for a variety of liver-related disorders and imbalances. Remember, we're now in the "practical" half of this book, so this information is useless unless you actually APPLY it!

First of all, here is an overview of signs and symptoms which might mean that your liver system is under stress or not functioning properly:

* Frequent headaches not related to tension and stress in the neck and shoulders (from poor posture when sitting and studying for instance) or from eyestrain

* Ongoing menstrual problems

* Weak tendons, ligaments, and muscles

* Acne, psoriasis, and other skin problems

* Tenderness or pain in the liver area

* Emotional excess, especially anger and depression; moodiness

* Blurring of vision or red eyes

* Bitter taste in the mouth

If you experience any of these symptoms, I recommend consulting with a trained holistic health practitioner and receive a comprehensive dietary, lifestyle, and herbal program, though if symptoms are mild, self-treatment is often appropriate.

FATS AND OILS

One of the greatest dangers in the modern diet is the kinds and quantities of fats and oils we consume. This is particularly pertinent to the liver, as it is a major site where fats and oils accumulate and are processed. Recently, people have started to eat more unsaturated fats because of the bad press saturated fats have received concerning their role in heart disease, a major killer in industrial countries. Ironically, however, manufacturers are now touting foods containing only unsaturated fats as being healthy and natural when the truth may be, in switching from saturated to unsaturated fats, we are only trading heart disease for cancer, premature aging, excessive skin wrinkles, and liver damage.

How so? Well, it all relates to how oxygen affects fats and oils in the body. Oxygen is the key element in the basic metabolic process of oxidation, that is, burning up and breaking down nutrients and other molecules. Many of the body's chemical reactions depend upon oxygen as a sort of catalytic fuel. However, because oxygen is a very reactive element, it doesn't always stick to only helpful biochemical reactions; it can also create harmful reactions by oxidizing various susceptible substances. Unsaturated oils are highly prone to such dangerous oxidation due to their carbon-carbon double bonds, which are easily attacked by oxygen.

Oil that has been oxidized becomes rancid. It should never be eaten because doing so can lead to the creation of free radicals in the body. Free radicals are molecules that are highly reactive to certain parts of healthy cells, such as cell-wall components and even DNA. Modern medical researchers think that free radicals "attack" the body's cells and lead to widespread tissue damage (such as in the liver), thus accelerating the aging process. Indeed, there is a free-radical theory of aging, which holds that many signs of aging, such as loss of flexibility and function in the joints, skin, and even internal organs (especially the liver), are promoted by free radicals.

Now about 17% of our total oxygen consumption turns into free radicals (Levine & Kidd, 1985) that can damage lipids and other cellular molecules. Most oxygen-consuming organisms have evolved defense systems to keep such free-radical damage to tolerable levels (Quintahilha, 1985). In human beings, these natural defense mechanisms include enzyme systems, such as the glutathione (GSH-T) peroxidase system we discussed earlier; naturally-occurring antioxidants such as vitamin C, A, and especially E; and DNA repair mechanisms. Nonetheless, these natural defense mechanisms did not evolve with the modern diet in mind, so they may need to be supplemented with healing plants that provide many of the essential elements needed to sustain them.

Having said this much about the under-publicized dangers of unsaturated oil, I must turn around and emphasize that unsaturated oils are not all bad. On the contrary, highly unsaturated fatty acids (such as linoleic acid), are crucial for human health—in moderate doses and preferably unheated. If you avoid junk and snack foods, eat a diet rich in whole, unprocessed foods, and take herbs and/or other supplements that contain antioxidants, you are in no danger of getting too much unsaturated oil.

Here are some general recommendations regarding oils and fats:

- Olive oil (extra virgin) is the most natural to our bodies, is resistant to oxidation, and contains a good balance of saturated, monosaturated (oleic), and unsaturated fatty acids (linoleic and linolenic). Oleic acid is less affected by oxygen and has been shown in a number of recent studies to benefit the heart and cardiovascular system.

- Linseed oil provides a rich source of essential fatty, linoleic, and linolenic acids.

- Avoid margarine, which contains oils that have been heated and pressurized to change their molecular structure—a biochemical nightmare for the body, especially for the liver. (Crisco is unmentionable).

- Lightly salted raw butter is superior to margarine. Where no refrigeration is available, ghee (clarified butter) can be used, because it won't rot (this is why it is used in India).

- Unsaturated oils (such as sunflower and safflower) should be tasted for rancidity (a sharp, biting taste). They should be stored in the refrigerator once opened.

• As much as possible, obtain essential fatty acids and other oils the body needs from whole nuts and seeds, preferably raw and organically grown.

Table 2 gives the percentage composition of saturated and unsaturated fatty acids in several common nuts, seeds, fats, and oils.

TABLE 2

Fatty Acid Composition of Common Nuts, Seeds, Fats, and Oils (Sources: Erasmus, Ensminger, et al.)

SOURCE	TOTAL FAT	SATURATED FAT	OLEIC	TOTAL UNSATURATED FAT
Nuts, Seeds	gms/100 gms			
Almonds	54.2	8%	67%	19%
Brazil nuts	66.9	26%	33%	38%
Cashew nuts	45.7	20%	57%	17%
Filberts	62.4	7%	80%	11%
Peanuts	48.7	17%	48%	24%
Sunflower	47.3	13%	19%	64%
Walnuts, English	64.0	11%	15%	66%
Fats, Oils				
Butter (81% fat)	—	62%	25%	4%
Corn oil	—	17%	24%	59%
Cottonseed oil	—	26%	18%	52%
Lard	—	40%	41%	15%
Linseed oil (flax)	—	9%	19%	72%
Olive oil	—	16%	76%	8%
Palm kernel	—	85%	13%	2%
Peanut oil	—	18%	47%	29%
Rape seed oil	—	7%	50%	37%
Salmon (7.4% fat)	—	18%	18%	39%
Sesame oil	—	13%	42%	45%
Soy bean oil	—	15%	26%	59%

BITTER TONICS, OR "BITTERS"

In the traditional medicine of both Europe and China, bitter herbs are thought to tonify and strengthen the digestive, immune, and nervous systems. Bitter tonic formulas, often called "bitters," usually contain bitter herbs like gentian, golden seal, artichoke, angelica, or blessed thistle, plus some aromatic or spicy herbs (ginger, fennel, or cardamon) to help counteract the formula's ability to cool and contract the digestive tract in some people. Many ready-made bitter formulas are available in natural food stores, and even in grocery stores and liquor stores (angostura bitters), though when they come from the latter two sources they must be checked for sugar and other undesirable additives.

Bitters are still used extensively in many cultures to strengthen digestion. In Europe, for example, "bitters cafes" are a popular social stop on the way home from work to prime the digestive tract for the evening meal. European naturopaths regularly recommend bitter wild greens or small doses of unripe fruit (such as green apples) to increase digestive powers. When I traveled in Greece recently, I was delighted to discover that people there customarily eat small, unripe, sour and bitter plums before meals. The Greeks also like to begin major meals with wild chicory greens, which are known to contain mild bitter principles that activate the digestive juices.

The traditional use of bitters makes good scientific sense, since by reflexive nerve action the bitter flavor immediately activates the secretion of gastric juices and tonifies the muscles of the digestive tract. Research has shown that bitters also activate the

Saturated vs. Unsaturated Oils

Both animal and vegetable oils and fats are made up of molecules called fatty acids, of which there are three main kinds—saturated, unsaturated, and monosaturated. Saturated fatty acids have more hydrogen atoms and less carbon-carbon double bonds than unsaturated fatty acids. Saturated fatty acids are usually solid at room temperature, like lard. Unsaturated fatty acids have less hydrogen atoms and more carbon-carbon double bonds. They are often liquid at room temperature, like soy oil. Monosaturated fatty acids have characteristics of both types and may be liquid at room temperature and solid when refrigerated, like olive oil, which contains mostly unsaturated and monosaturated fatty acids.

Although there is still much to learn about the way the body responds to a constant diet of certain kinds of fats, recent research strongly supports the idea that fresh, cold-processed oils which contain mostly unsaturated or monosaturated fatty acids are far preferable to oils that are refined, heated, and made up of mostly saturated fatty acids (like animal fat). It is important to note, however, that even unsaturated oils may be unhealthful if they have been heated or exposed to air for a long time, because then they lead to the formation of free radicals in the body. Most snack foods such as chips, crackers, cookies, etc., as well as many other foods commonly sold in supermarkets, now contain heated, oxidized, unsaturated oils. These foods should therefore be avoided. A recent Japanese study notes that liver damage due to oxidized oils in food now has to be regarded as a serious problem for human health (Kiso, 1987).

parasympathetic nervous system (which "controls" the digestive tract), as well as the immune system (Maiwald, 1987). Indeed, some bitter compounds, such as the amarogentin in the herb gentian, are so powerfully bitter that they can be detected in a dilution of 1:50,000!

HOW TO TAKE BITTERS

It is important to understand that bitters must be taken over a period of weeks or months before their full effect is achieved. Taking them for a day or two might bestow some benefits, but 90% of the effect builds slowly.

Bitter formulas are taken 1/2 hour to 15 minutes before a meal, or just after eating. Take 1/2 to 1 teaspoon of the liquid extract; 1-2 teaspoons of a bitters tea (drink it at room temperature, not hot); or 1 dropperful of a more concentrated formula. Note that some commercial bitters also contain a mild laxative herb such as aloe or senna. These should be avoided by people who have diarrhea or loose bowels. I have also found that these formulas may not agree with people who lack vital energy.

Here's a recipe for making homemade bitters.

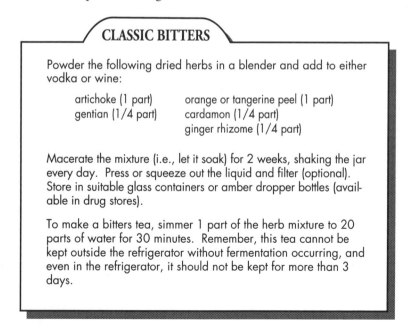

CLASSIC BITTERS

Powder the following dried herbs in a blender and add to either vodka or wine:

artichoke (1 part)   orange or tangerine peel (1 part)
gentian (1/4 part)   cardamon (1/4 part)
                            ginger rhizome (1/4 part)

Macerate the mixture (i.e., let it soak) for 2 weeks, shaking the jar every day. Press or squeeze out the liquid and filter (optional). Store in suitable glass containers or amber dropper bottles (available in drug stores).

To make a bitters tea, simmer 1 part of the herb mixture to 20 parts of water for 30 minutes. Remember, this tea cannot be kept outside the refrigerator without fermentation occurring, and even in the refrigerator, it should not be kept for more than 3 days.

OTHER DIETARY FACTORS

Following is a short list of other dietary factors to consider when you are trying to eat for optimal liver health. Table 3 summarizes handy dietary sources of substances that build, protect, and/or cleanse the liver.

- Protein: both too little or too much can disrupt liver enzymes. About 35 to 60 grams/day is optimal. Most people in industrialized countries eat far too much protein. When bacteria in the large intestine act on protein residues, toxins are produced that may be absorbed into the bloodstream.

- Sulfur-containing foods such as cabbage, brussels sprouts, broccoli, nuts, and seeds, are potent enzyme-builders. Take at least one serving a day of these foods—especially of vegetables from the mustard family, which provide excellent enzyme support for the liver.

- Fats are difficult for the liver to process, yet they provide a good energy source. A small amount of unsaturated fat is essential to health, but excess will oxidize easily, leading to the formation of potentially harmful free radicals.

- Protectors such as vitamins, minerals, herbs, amino acids, and flavonoids, should be present in ample amounts. Live vegetable juices (carrot, beet, celery, or parsley) are recommended. Or take a complete nutritional system supplement.

- Refined sugars, such as glucose, can lower enzyme activity. Sweet foods can be a healthful addition to the diet if they contain predominantly complex and unrefined sugars, such as those found in all fruits, vegetables, whole grains, and in barley malt and rice syrup. For a sweeter treat, use more concentrated sugars such as dates, dried fruit, pure unrefined cane sugar, and honey in moderation.

- Phosphatidyl choline is a constituent of lecithin that can improve the health of the microsomal membrane (in the liver) where enzymes are produced. Soybean products are a good source for this substance, as is commercially available lecithin.

TABLE 3.

DIETARY SOURCES OF LIVER BUILDERS, CLEANSERS, AND PROTECTORS

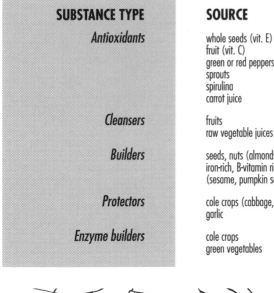

SUBSTANCE TYPE	SOURCE
Antioxidants	whole seeds (vit. E) fruit (vit. C) green or red peppers (vit. A) sprouts spirulina carrot juice
Cleansers	fruits raw vegetable juices
Builders	seeds, nuts (almonds) iron-rich, B-vitamin rich foods (sesame, pumpkin seeds; millet)
Protectors	cole crops (cabbage, broccoli) garlic
Enzyme builders	cole crops green vegetables

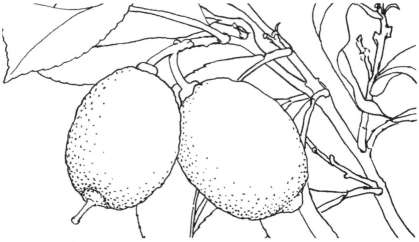

Lemon
Citrus limon

HERBAL THERAPY

In this section I will discuss various types of herbal remedies for liver disorders. Liver and gallbladder "flushes" are useful for a wide range of imbalances. Specific herbs and herbal formulas, on the other hand, need to be selected according to a person's condition and constitution.

THE LIVER FLUSH

Liver flushes are used to stimulate elimination of wastes from the body, to open and cool the liver, to increase bile flow, and to improve overall liver functioning. They also help purify the blood and the lymph. I have taken liver flushes for many years now and can heartily recommend them. And if you make the herbal formula right, it can be quite tasty. Here's how to make a liver flush:

1. Mix any fresh-squeezed citrus juices together to make 1 cup of liquid. Orange and grapefruit juices are good, but always mix in some lemon or lime. The final mix should have a sour taste—the more sour, the more cleansing and activating. This mixture can be watered down to taste with spring or distilled water.

2. Add 1-2 cloves of fresh-squeezed garlic, plus a small amount of fresh ginger juice, which you can obtain by grating ginger on a cheese or vegetable grater and then pressing the resulting fibers in a garlic press. (Note: Both garlic and ginger have shown amazing liver-protective qualities in recent studies (Hikino, 1986). Garlic contains strong antioxidant principles and also provides important sulfur compounds that the liver uses to build certain enzymes.)

3. Mix in 1 tablespoon of high-quality olive oil, blend (or shake well in a glass container), and drink.

4. Follow the liver flush with two cups of cleansing herbal tea. I like "Polari-Tea", which consists of the herbs below. I make plenty of this tea and keep it in quart canning jars or juice bottles, so it is always available.

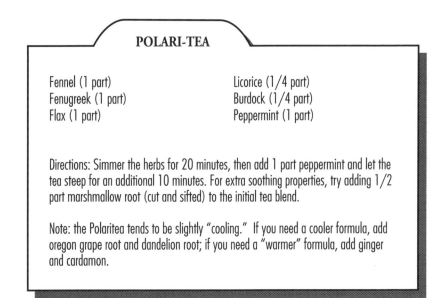

POLARI-TEA

Fennel (1 part)
Fenugreek (1 part)
Flax (1 part)

Licorice (1/4 part)
Burdock (1/4 part)
Peppermint (1 part)

Directions: Simmer the herbs for 20 minutes, then add 1 part peppermint and let the tea steep for an additional 10 minutes. For extra soothing properties, try adding 1/2 part marshmallow root (cut and sifted) to the initial tea blend.

Note: the Polaritea tends to be slightly "cooling." If you need a cooler formula, add oregon grape root and dandelion root; if you need a "warmer" formula, add ginger and cardamon.

5. Drink the liver flush in the morning (preferably after some stretching and breathing exercises), then do not eat any other food for one hour.

When and how often should one take liver flushes? I usually do two full cycles of 10 days on, 3 days off in the spring and again in the fall, with a 3-day rest between each cycle. However, I know many people who benefit from a single 10-day flush once at each equinox time. In any case, though, if one really feels a need for a liver flush, any time is the right time. I have never seen anyone experience negative side effects from this procedure.

There are also several good commercial formulas for liver-cleansing available in natural food stores everywhere, both in bulk and in tea-bag form. One product I can recommend is a blend called "Puri-Tea," from herbalist Brigitte Mars. It contains peppermint, red clover, fennel, licorice, cleavers, dandelion, Oregon grape, burdock root, butternut bark, chickweed, parsley root, and nettles.

If you want more cleansing action than simple teas or formulas provide, try adding a fast with fresh fruit and vegetable juices. You can also take an enema each day. A good enema can be made by adding the juice of 1/2 of a lemon to 1 quart of tepid water (lemon-water in general is a good cleanser because citric and other plant acids in lemon juice can chelate, or bind

• SAVES TIME: Hours a day are often spent in working to pay for food, shopping, preparing food, eating, and cleaning up the kitchen.

• REST: Give your digestive system a much-needed rest.

• INCREASES ENERGY: Tremendous amounts of vital energy usually spent in digestion, assimilation, and elimination are saved for other purposes, instead.

• SPIRITUAL UPLIFTMENT: All great spiritual figures have fasted. Fasting helps cut our attachment to the physical world.

• CLEANSING: The body is very wise. When it can't get energy from food, it breaks down diseased and second-rate or toxic cells, recycles the usable components, and eliminates wastes.

• LOSE WEIGHT: Not eating is one of the fastest ways to lose excess weight. Fat is broken down before muscle tissue in the fasting process.

• HEALING: Even intractable diseases have been healed during fasts (see the Appendix for this).

• BREAKS ADDICTIONS: Fasting is one of the very best ways to break addictions. It can strengthen discrimination and will power. After a fast, the last thing you want to do is smoke a cigarette or drink coffee or alcohol. Many years ago, I broke my seemingly unbreakable addiction to tobacco with a fast.

• APPRECIATION: In no period of human history has such a variety of food been as readily available as today. There is so much abundance that it is easy to even become blasé about delicacies such as tropical fruits and artichoke hearts. Fasting helps us realize just how blessed we really are. I still vividly remember how delicious a bite of apple tasted after my first 2-week fast. The finest ambrosia of the Gods couldn't be better!

with, and remove heavy metals and other toxic wastes accumulated in the body). Retain for 10 to 15 minutes (if possible), apply clockwise lower abdominal massage, then expel.

For complete cleansing and fasting programs, see my book *Foundations of Health*.

THE GALLBLADDER FLUSH

Please note: This technique is for people who have had previous experience with cleansing programs and have practiced a predominantly whole foods diet for some time.

The gallbladder flush is useful for people who are experienced with fasting and cleansing and who want to go a step further and remove even more old wastes stored in liver cells and other tissues. This flush should not be used more than once a year. I have seen some people become nauseated after drinking the flush, but nothing worse than that.

1. About an hour before bedtime, drink 1/4 cup of extra virgin olive oil, followed by 1/4 cup of mixed, fresh-squeezed citrus juices (50% grapefruit juice, 25% lemon juice, and 25% orange juice). Repeat this process every 15 minutes for an hour, so that you drink a total of 1 cup of olive oil and 1 cup of citrus juice.

2. After the drinks, go to bed, making sure to lie on your right side. By tradition, this is thought to allow the oil to be discharged from the gallbladder more efficiently, but whether this is in fact true has not been proven as far as I know.

3. In the morning, take an enema consisting of 1 quart of warm distilled water with the addition of the juice of 1/2 lemon.

Note: It is often good to combine the gallbladder flush with a 3- or 7-day juice fast. Toxic wastes released during fasting will be effectively eliminated during the strong bile flush and enema.

The purpose of this flush is to strongly activate the liver and gallbladder. When the liver encounters so much oil, it reacts by producing a large amount of bile, which the gallbladder then squirts into the intestines. It is thought that such a strong flow of bile will carry with it deeply stored toxins which are then flushed out of the body with the enema. Activating the liver and gallbladder so strongly may also run them through a thorough drill, thus strengthening them.

During the enema, watch for little green "stones" or marbles that may be eliminated. I have heard these called gallstones, but they are probably saponified oil. At any rate, my own

3-DAY JUICE FAST

For a novice faster, I usually recommend a short 3-day fast using fruit juices. Water fasts usually are too severe for most people, and are probably not the best kind of fast for today's world of industrial chemicals and heavy metals that may be stored in our bodies. Besides, fruit juices contain pectin and other purifying substances that help remove toxic wastes.

Always eat raw fruits and vegetables for two or three days before and after the fast, to ease in and out of the fasting period. During the fast, drink nothing but water and freshly-extracted juices. If fresh juice is impossible to obtain during the fast, then use bottled organic grape or apple juice diluted in a 1:1 ratio with distilled water. However, even fresh-squeezed grapefruit juice and distilled water is preferable to bottled juices, because the body responds best to the vitality of fresh juice. Note that the whole process actually lasts 10 days counting preparation and transition to a normal diet.

My usual program for a 3-day fast is as follows:

Days 1-3 (Preparation): Upon rising, do 20-30 minutes of deep breathing and stretching (continue this throughout the fast). Then drink a liver flush as detailed on p. 23. Follow with two cups of cleansing tea. Eat raw fruits and vegetables, salads, whole apples, pears, grapefruit—but not bananas (juicy foods only). Drink as much distilled water with fresh lemon juice added to taste as desired. More herbal tea in the evening is optional.

Days 4-6 (The Fast): Start each day during the actual fast with the liver flush and tea, and follow one or two hours later with about 6-8 ounces of freshly-squeezed fruit juice (usually apple, grape or grapefruit) diluted with distilled water in a 1:1 ratio. A few hours later, try 6-8

ounces of mixed vegetable juice, usually a combination of organic carrot and celery with a touch of beet or parsley. In the evening take another glass of fruit juice, and perhaps a cup of herb tea. Finally, before bed take an enema consisting of 1 quart of warm distilled water mixed with the juice of 1/2 lemon. If you've never taken an enema before, you will be surprised at how much comes out. (Remember that during a fast the bowels will usually cease to move.) This will get out any waste material that is being eliminated into the colon and will also soften and remove old fecal matter that may be hanging onto the walls of the colon.

On the last day of the fast, I usually go to a professional for a colonic flush. This ensures that my colon is thoroughly cleaned. During the colonic, I am always amazed at what I see come out—even after fasting and taking enemas. Some people prefer to have a series of two or three colonics after a fast.

Day 8: I always break a 3-day fast with a raw salad, according to Paul Bragg's instructions. Paul Bragg was my health teacher—see his book *The Miracle of Fasting*—I highly recommend it. I have tried different ways to break a short fast and have found this way the most satisfactory. The roughage in the salad helps move the bowels and acts as a sort of "broom" to sweep out further wastes. My first salad consists of grated cabbage, carrot, finely chopped celery, a little grated beet root, and perhaps some finely shredded romaine lettuce. I eat a good-sized bowl of this salad at about noon of the day after the 3-day fast (the 8th day overall). In the evening I eat more raw vegetables, or a little vegetable broth, depending on how I am feeling.

experience with the flush, plus my observation of others who have done it, have convinced me that old, negative emotions can be effectively eliminated during the process. Anger and frustration, especially, are purged. It is possible that one may experience strange feelings during the process, as if some drug were floating around in the blood stream. This may be due to old drug residues being re-experienced as they are eliminated from the body—or it may be due to a systemic hormonal reaction to all the oil. I tend to believe the former theory, but no definitive tests have been done to prove which view is right.

HERBAL REMEDIES

In scientific terms, herbs contain several kinds of substances that protect and fortify the liver. These fall into five classes:

1. Antioxidants (protect cells and tissues in the liver)

2. Membrane stabilizing compounds (protect liver-cell integrity)

3. Choleretics (promote bile; help detoxify the liver)

4. Substances that prevent depletion of certain vital sulfur compounds

5. Substances that either stimulate or reduce the activity of liver enzyme systems

Natural Liver Therapy

Table 5 lists some herbal sources of these five types of substances. You will note that vitamins, minerals, amino acids, and flavonoids also have these five different properties, so I have listed them under the herbs. Although many of these vitamins, minerals, and amino acids are available in synthetic supplements, I recommend obtaining them directly from herbs and foods, because plants contain these substances in more easily assimilable forms. Also, synthetic supplements may interfere with the uptake and utilization of other vital elements in your diet. Another advantage of natural over synthetic sources is that herbs are an excellent source of flavonoids, which are coloring pigments in plants that can strengthen blood vessels, act as antioxidants, and have other beneficial effects as well (for instance, they accumulate under the skin and protect it from ultra-violet radiation as well as reducing inflammation in the body.) And last, but not least, recent studies show that herbs have enzyme-modifying effects and provide structural elements for some enzymes (Chang, et al., 1985)

Synthetic supplements, on the other hand, neither contain nor promote the activity of enzymes, those all-important catalysts in the process of digestion.

Day 9: Eat fruits and vegetables during the day, with the addition of a steamed potato or other steamed green vegetables.

Day 10: Begin to eat regularly, but lightly. Chew each bite well and combine foods carefully. I always find that by this time I desire no processed foods. It feels so good to have had the discipline and wisdom to fast that I don't want to put anything in my body that is not the very best fresh, organic food.

Suggestions:

I have never seen any serious problems during a fast, but it is common to experience symptoms such as:

- dizziness
- mild heart palpitations
- weakness
- light headedness
- tiredness
- forgetfulness
- mild nausea
- a bad taste in the mouth, known as "faster's breath"
- a gnawing or empty feeling in the stomach and abdomen

If these become frightening or unpleasant, you can slow down the cleansing process by using a juice or broth that is less cleansing for a short time, until the symptoms abate. Also, it always helps to rest, if possible, and to focus on the positive aspects of the cleansing and healing process. Envision the wastes leaving your body. I often imagine a pure mountain meadow filled with wildflowers and with a crystal clear stream flowing through it. I imagine myself bathing in the pristine water, and I think of all wastes leaving me and returning to mother earth, where they are broken down into pure elemental components.

Natural Liver Therapy

TABLE 5.

SOURCES OF LIVER-PROTECTING SUBSTANCES

ANTIOXIDANTS	STABILIZING	CHOLERETICS	SOURCE OF SULFUR	PROMOTES ENZYMES
Plant Sources				
artichoke		artichoke		
bilberry				
cabbage	cabbage		cabbage	cabbage
capillaris		capillaris		
cayenne				
		dandelion		
garlic		garlic	garlic	
ginkgo				
lemon balm				
licorice				
milk thistle	milk thistle			milk thistle
rosemary				
schisandra				schisandra
skullcap				
turmeric				
Vitamins				
C				
E				
A				
Minerals				
zinc				
selenium				
Amino Acids				
methionine			methionine	
glutathione				
cysteine			cysteine	
Flavonoids				
catechin				
quercetin				
rutin				
kaempferol				
luteolin				

This table (Table 5) is designed to give you an overview of some of the active ingredients in foods and herbs that can benefit the liver. In actual practice, many herbs are taken in combinations called formulas. A number of formulas I have found to be helpful for specific liver-related ailments can be found starting on page 39. You can also design your own formulas by blending several herbs together and trying the blend out for taste and effectiveness.

Remember to start out with a small dose (1 cup/day of a tea) to check for individual sensitivity before going up to a full therapeutic dose (about 3 cups of tea per day—1 cup morning, afternoon, and evening). Or simply select a good quality ready-made product (ask your supplement department consultant) available in natural food stores and try a bottle. It is good to follow a supplement program for up to 3 months to give it a fair trial, though you should start seeing results within 2 weeks.

When designing programs, keep in mind that herbs are usually blended together based on their "energetics." This means that some herbs are stimulating (cleansing, cooling, or warming), some are tonifying (strengthening), and some are protective. Generally, if you are weak and run-down, add tonifying herbs to specific herbs that sound right for your condition. If you are not particularly run-down or chronically fatigued, you might try a mild cleansing program with the specific herbs. If you feel hot, or have signs or symptoms of pathogenic (related to illness or symptoms) heat, add cooling herbs (most bitter herbs and formulas are cooling); if you feel cold and your digestion is particularly sluggish, try a warming formula, such as an Indian spice tea (ginger, cardamon, cinnamon, clove, etc.). A full discussion of formulating is beyond the scope of this present book, but more information can be found in my *Foundations of Health*.

Here is a short list of commonly used liver herbs classified according to this energetic system:

Strong Cleansers	Gentle Cleansers	Builders	Protectors
cascara	artichoke	milk thistle	schisandra
butternut	burdock	astragalus	garlic
dock	dandelion root	oat	milk thistle
	Oregon grape root		turmeric

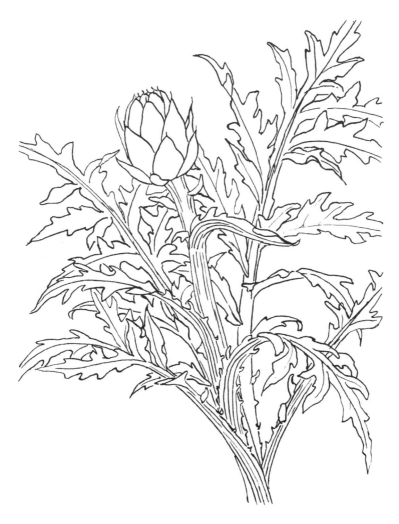

Artichoke
Cynara scolymus

Another thing herbalists consider is whether an herb has a cool, neutral, or warm energy, since this will determine what types of conditions it can be used for. For example, if a patient has symptoms of liver "fire" (headaches, red face, anger, high blood pressure, etc.), a cooling herb would be useful while a warming one might even be harmful. On the other a hand, for a person suffering from liver stagnation (headaches, belching, depression, anger, etc.), a warming herb might be beneficial. Herbal formulas that take

TABLE 6

SYNDROME	SIGNS & SYMPTOMS	WESTERN CORRELATION
Stagnant liver chi	depression, anger, frustration; lumps in neck, breast, etc.; poor digestion	congested liver; insufficient blood & oxygen
Deficient liver yin	dizziness, eye problems, flushed face, irritability, ringing in the ears, warm palms and soles	enzymes deficient, low vital energy, adrenal weakness
Blazing liver fire/ liver fire rising	hypertension, migraine, dizziness, red face and eyes, insomnia, violent anger, bitter taste in the mouth	acute conjunctivitis, excess hormones, liver too metabolically active
Liver blood deficiency/ poor blood storage	weak tendons and ligaments, poor digestion, chronic menstrual problems, scanty menstruation	liver overworked, anemia, deficient blood
Liver wind moving/ stagnancy in outer body with overheated liver creates wind;	rigid body, vertigo, extreme dizziness, severe pain, convulsions, spasms, tremor	differential temperature gradient: hypertension, stroke, epilepsy, coldness
Damp heat invasion of the liver	liver tenderness, enlargement, yellow eyes, dark yellow urine, light stools (jaundice)	hepatitis, jaundice, inflammation of the gall bladder

Natural Liver Therapy

all of these factors into consideration are presented in the next section, where specific liver-related complaints are discussed.

Table 6 presents the major liver syndromes as they are differentiated and diagnosed in Traditional Chinese Medicine (TCM). I've also included modern, Western correlations for these syndromes, plus a short list of herbs commonly used for them. TCM theory is especially useful because it is so highly articulated, having been refined and tested for thousands of years.

MAJOR LIVER SYNDROMES IN TCM

THERAPY	HERBS
dredge liver, smooth chi, promote bile flow	Use dry, fragrant herbs: burdock, Cyperus, dandelion, milk thistle
tonify the yin, pacify the liver, subdue the yang, clear heat	Use sweet, moist, bitter, and cooling herbs: rehmannia, lycium berries, Tribulus, peony, margarita shell
clear liver, purge fire	Use cool, bitter herbs: gentian, chrysanthemum, skullcap
tonify blood, nurture & clear liver	Use neutral, biting herbs: lycii berries, rehmannia, dong quai, fo-ti (he shou wu), mulberry fruit (sang shen), longan
pacify liver, extinguish wind, remove temperature gradient by circulating blood and energy	gastrodia and gastrodia formulas (tian ma pien); valerian, skullcap with yerba mansa or calamus root
remove dampness and heat from the liver	dandelion, milk thistle, turmeric, artichoke, gentian; Chinese patent, Lung Tan

Tables 7 and 8 present other herbs that may be used for liver and gallbladder disorders and give their actions according to both Chinese and traditional Western herbalism. Note that there are no herbs specifically for the gallbladder, while there are herbs just for the liver. However, the double-action herbs for liver and gallbladder together are especially stimulating to the bile and the health of gallbladder. Although I realize that many lay readers will not be able to use this information to design their own herbal formulas, I have included these tables for natural health practitioners and students of herbalism.

PROGRAMS FOR SPECIFIC COMPLAINTS

In this last section, I will give complete instructions for recognizing and remedying a variety of liver-related disorders and complaints. I have experimented with these herbal formulas and natural therapies for over 20 years, and I have found them to be highly effective for a great number of people, including myself. It is important to understand that herbs alone may not counteract the negative consequences of continuing bad habits. To achieve a state of optimum health, you must combine herbal treatment with proper diet, various other natural therapies, and a lifestyle that has a time and place for relaxation. Again, if your liver-related condition is serious, or if your symptoms are confusing and you are not sure which of the following programs applies to you, I recommend that you seek the help of a qualified health practitioner.

A word on making herbal teas: for flowers, leaves, and other light parts of a plant, make an infusion. This is done by bringing water to a boil, taking it off the heat, adding the herbs, and then covering the pot and letting the mixture steep for 10-20 minutes. For heavier herb parts, such as the roots, bark, or seeds, a decoction is preferable. To make a decoction, simmer the herbs for 20-60 minutes.

To judge how much herb to add to a measured amount of water, use the general formula of 1:10 (grams herb:milliliters water or ounces herb:ounces water) for decoctions and 1:20 for infusions. The ratio of herbs to water, as well as the length of time for infusing of decocting, can be varied according to need and taste. The longer an herb steeps, the stronger the tea.

Finally, it is best to prepare herbal teas in a stainless steel, glass, ceramic, or clay pot. Strictly avoid teflon-coated pans and aluminum. Herbalists

TABLE 7.

HERBS FOR THE LIVER AND GALLBLADDER

GENUS	COMMON NAME	CHINESE ENERGY	ACTION	WESTERN ACTION
Achillea	yarrow	neutral	purges fire	anti-inflammatory, decongesting, diaphoretic
Allium	garlic	warm	dredges liver	warms & opens liver, stimulates bile
Anemone	hepatica	cold	pacifies liver	soothes liver, tonic
Antennaria	pussy paws	warm	-	deobstruent
Arctium	burdock	cold	purges fire	stimulates bile, protects, tonifies
Artemisia vulgaris	mugwort	neutral	dispels wind	for jaundice; opens liver
Artemisia capillaris	capillaris	cool	cools fire	stimulates bile
Avena	wild oat	neutral	-	improves nerve tone; nutritive tonic, anti-addictive
Berberis	Oregon grape rt.	cold	purges fire	anti-inflammatory; opens liver, stimulates bile, benefits acne
Centaurium	centaury	cold	clears damp heat	cleansing, tonic, improves protein digestion
Chelidonium	celandine	cool	dredges liver	removes bile stones, increases phagocytosis
Cichorium	chicory	cool	dredges, cools	deobstruent; opens & tonifies
Cnicus	blessed thistle	cool	dredges, cools	stimulates bile; opens & cools
Cynara	artichoke	cool	dredges, cools	stimulates bile; opens & regenerates
Gentiana	gentian	cool	clears damp	stimulates bile; opens & cools liver fire, activates immune function
Inula	elecampane	warm	subdues yang	resolves phlegm in the lung, warms liver
Lavandula	lavender	cool	-	lifts spirits, calms emotions
Raphanus	wild radish	neutral	-	digestive tonic, removes mucus
Rosmarinus	rosemary	cool	-	warms surface, dispels wind, energy stimulant, antioxidant, liver protector
Silybum	milk thistle	neutral	yin tonic	regenerates, protects the liver, detoxifies; antioxidant
Taraxacum	dandelion	cool	dredge, cool	deobstruent; opens, cools liver fire

Natural Liver Therapy

TABLE 8.

HERBS FOR THE LIVER

GENUS	COMMON NAME	TCM* TEMP.	TCM* ACTION	WESTERN ACTION
Angelica	angelica	warm	moistens yin	nourishes, activates blood
Atractylodes	cang zhu	warm	activates blood	protects liver; improves digestion
Berberis	Oregon grape	cold	purges fire	anti-inflammatory; cools liver
Bryonia	bryony	warm	-	acrid irritant; stimulates liver
Ceanothus	red root	cool	clears damp, heat	anti-inflammatory; cleanses lymph
Chionanthus	fringe tree	cool	subdues yang	for jaundice & bile obstructions, general tonic and adaptogen
Coptis	gold thread	cold	purges fire	anti-inflammatory; detoxifies & dries
Coriolus	polypore	neutral	moistens yin	moistens, increases phagocytosis, supports immune function
Cucurma	turmeric	warm	invigorates blood	protects liver, reduces inflammation
Dioscorea	wild yam	neutral	supports stomach/spleen	balances hormones, nourishes
Galium	cleavers	cool	clears damp heat	diuretic, removes wastes, relieves lymph congestion
Glycyrrhiza	licorice	neutral	clears heat	protects liver, antiinflammatory
Hydrastis	golden seal	cold	purges fire	anti-inflammatory; opens liver, stimulates bile, slightly toxic
Iris	blue flag	hot	acrid stimulant	warms surface, removes congestion
Larrea	chaparral	warm	-	warms surface, detoxifies, deobstruent
Leptandra	black root	warm	dredges liver	stimulates liver, bile, glands
Linaria	toad flax	warm	dredges liver	for jaundice & skin disease
Picraena	quassia	warm	-	small dose regenerates & tonifies
Plantago	plantain seed	cold	drains damp	protects liver; anti-diarrheal, antibacterial
Rhamnus	cascara	cool	dispels heat	bowel stimulant, laxative clears liver congestion, heat
Salvia	dan shen	cool	moves blood	removes liver scarring, reduces pain
Sanguinaria	bloodroot	acrid, cool	-	warms surface & mucosa; stim. bile, attacks tumors
Schisandra	five flavors berry	warm	supports yin	protects liver; adaptogenic
Scutellaria	skullcap	cold	removes heat	subdues liver yang, protects liver
Xanthoxylum	prickly ash	warm	-	deobstruent, moves blood, relieves pain

*TCM = Traditional Chinese Medicine

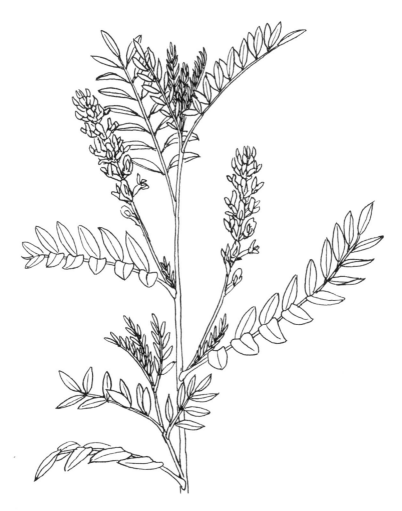

Licorice
Glycyrrhiza glabra

agree that the latter may act as a source of potentially toxic substances or affect the tea's energetic properties.

POOR DIGESTION
(CONGESTED, OVERWORKED LIVER)

Diagnostic symptoms: Soreness in the liver area under moderate fingertip pressure; painful digestion; gas pains; constipation (less than 1 bowel movement per day); feeling of fullness in stomach and intestines; loss of appetite; PMS; depression; marked distaste for oily foods.

Dietary recommendations: Rest the digestive tract and liver by allowing at least 12 hours between the evening and morning meals. After 7 p.m., eat only small portions of fruit or drink herb tea. Exercise or do some physical work in the morning before eating breakfast. A moderate walk after a large meal will help stimulate the digestive juices. Do not overeat. Try skipping a meal (lunch), and eat light, easily digested foods such as steamed vegetables and raw salad greens (make some of these bitter). Eat semi-sweet fruits such as apples and pears in moderation. Add olive oil to food in teaspoonful doses and go easy on cooked or refined oils.

Do the liver flush (see page 23 for instructions) for 1 week on, 2 days off, and 1 week on. This cycle can be repeated for 1 month, but not more than 2 months. Enemas are of some benefit when there is a history of heavy, refined foods in the diet.

Herbal recommendations: Take herbs that decongest the liver, increase blood flow, and have an opening, slightly warming action. I recommend the following basic formula:

Remember, this is a strong medicinal blend, and as with all such formulas, it is best to start with small doses—perhaps only several tablespoons per dose at first. Then work up to the full recommended dose after a few days, being sure to check for individual sensitivities and reactions as you go. Note that if your condition is mild, this tea is not for you; drink "Polari-Tea" or "Puri-Tea" instead (again, see the section on liver flushes, page 23). Both of these are milder, taste better, and can be taken several times a day, or as desired.

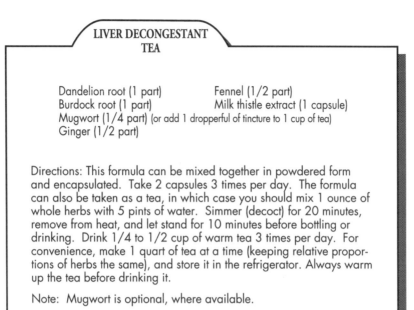

LIVER DECONGESTANT TEA

Dandelion root (1 part)   Fennel (1/2 part)
Burdock root (1 part)   Milk thistle extract (1 capsule)
Mugwort (1/4 part) (or add 1 dropperful of tincture to 1 cup of tea)
Ginger (1/2 part)

Directions: This formula can be mixed together in powdered form and encapsulated. Take 2 capsules 3 times per day. The formula can also be taken as a tea, in which case you should mix 1 ounce of whole herbs with 5 pints of water. Simmer (decoct) for 20 minutes, remove from heat, and let stand for 10 minutes before bottling or drinking. Drink 1/4 to 1/2 cup of warm tea 3 times per day. For convenience, make 1 quart of tea at a time (keeping relative proportions of herbs the same), and store it in the refrigerator. Always warm up the tea before drinking it.

Note: Mugwort is optional, where available.

Other natural therapies: Massage the liver area by lying flat on your back and pressing your fingertips up under the right side of your rib cage. Use increasingly deep, circular motions, until all soreness or tightness is relieved (if soreness persists for more than a week, or if there is a pronounced tenderness in the area, it may be wise to seek the aid of a skilled natural health practitioner). Too much sitting and too little physical activity can block up the intestinal and liver area. It is good to massage this area often and to eat lightly until this condition improves.

I have also found that one of the most harmful influences on the liver and digestion is excessive thinking. Sitting and staring at a computer monitor all day is especially nefarious. Two of my greatest allies in balancing my own life in this regard are walking and meditation.

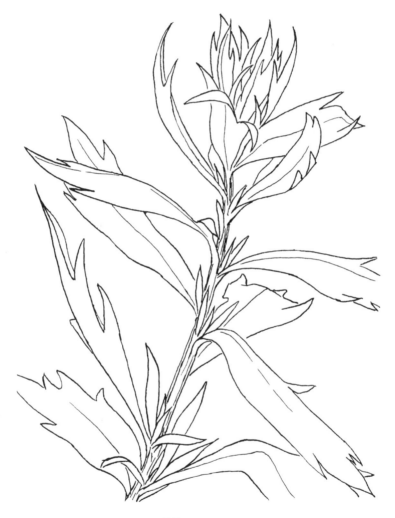

Mugwort
Artemesia vulgaris

POOR FAT DIGESTION

Diagnostic symptoms: Feeling of nausea or soreness in gut after fatty meals; burping with an oily taste in the mouth or throat; avoidance of or revulsion to fatty foods.

Dietary recommendations: Rest the digestive tract and take liver flushes, as explained above. One of the best and most obvious remedies is to avoid foods cooked or fried in oil. Keep diet mostly fresh—about 30% raw fruits and vegetables and 70% steamed vegetables, whole grains and either aduki or mung beans. Try using some white organic basmati rice instead of brown rice—it's easier to digest.

Herbal recommendations: Take herbs to increase bile flow, especially the following milk thistle/artichoke combination.

Other natural therapies: If nausea after fatty meals persists, it might be an indication of a deep-seated liver imbalance, in which case I recommend seeking the help of a skilled natural health practitioner.

PRO-BILE TEA

Milk thistle seed extract (1 part—1 dropperful or 1 tablet of the extract per cup)

> Artichoke leaves (1 part)
> Dandelion root (1 part)
> Mugwort (1/4 part)
> Yellow dock root powder (1/2 part)
> Peppermint leaf (1/2 part)
> Sweeten to taste with stevia herb

Directions: Warm the tea to room temperature and drink 1/4 to 1/2 cup of the tea before meals, especially fatty meals.

**Note: It is best to buy yellow dock as whole as possible, and powder it yourself in a coffee grinder or blender.

IRRITABLE BOWEL SYNDROME

Diagnostic symptoms: Burning or uncomfortable feelings in the bowels; alternating diarrhea and constipation; frequent gas and rumbling sounds in the intestines. These symptoms are usually worse after stress or when tired. There may be periods that are symptom-free, then times of pronounced symptoms. Bowel diseases or imbalances are extremely difficult to diagnose. Pains can move from one area of the abdomen to another. Other possible ailments showing similar symptoms include appendicitis, diverticulitis, microflora imbalance due to antibiotics or other chemical factors, gallstones, and even cancer. However, always remember that cancer is the least likely. Nonetheless, it is wise to consult a qualified health practitioner if symptoms are serious enough to go on for more than a week or 10 days.

Dietary recommendations: Feed the beneficial flora in your intestines with foods containing ample soluble and insoluble fiber. Such foods included lightly cooked apples and other fruits, steamed vegetables, and grains that are easy to digest and are usually non-allergenic (i.e., millet, buckwheat, corn, and especially rice). Half-refined white rice is easier to digest than brown rice. Take a good probiotics supplement with a variety of beneficial organisms, such as *Lactobacillus acidophilus, L. rhamnosus, L. bulgaricus, Bifidobacteria bifidum,* or *Streptococcus faecium.* Make your own rejuvelac, yogurt, or sauerkraut. See my book *Foundations of Health* for complete instructions, programs and recipes, as well as the most up to date information on probiotics.

Do not overeat or eat complex combinations—keep things simple. Sometimes several smaller meals during the day are easier to handle than one or two big ones. Also, eat most foods lightly to well-cooked, and avoid common allergenic foods such as wheat, dairy products (especially pasteurized dairy), and eggs.

Herbal recommendations: I have had excellent results using the high-mucilage tea below, "Herbal Slime Tea." Carry a quart jar with you and sip it throughout the day. Drink up to 1 quart a day (4 cups).

Other Recommendations: Be sure to follow the programs for promoting beneficial microflora recommended above. It is essential to maintain a healthy microflora in any kind of bowel ailment. Research is increasingly identifying disordered microflora as a cause or contributing factor in irritable bowel syndrome and related bowel imbalances.

HERBAL SLIME TEA

Flax seed (1 part)
Marshmallow root (1 part)
Licorice root (1/4 part)
Fenugreek (1 part)
Caraway seed (or Fennel) (1/4 part)

Directions: Simmer the ingredients in water for 40 minutes, then remove from heat and allow to steep for 15 minutes. Strain the tea and store it in the refrigerator in quart jars or other suitable containers. The tea can be used for up to 5 days, if kept cool. Drink the tea as often as possible. I carry my tea with me wherever I go sipping it or drinking a cup every hour or two.

GAS (FLATULENCE)

Diagnostic symptoms: A bloated feeling accompanied by various pains in the abdomen or side; frequent passing of gas. Gas pains usually come and go and are not exercise-related. In fact they may be relieved by movement. Applying pressure with the fingers to different abdominal areas will usually aggravate the pains. Note that gas pains can radiate into the lower chest cavity, mimicking a heart attack. If these symptoms persist, consult a qualified health practitioner.

Dietary recommendations: Keep food combinations simple. Sugars mixed with protein foods will often lead to gas. Soak legumes for one or two days before cooking. Pour off the soak water a few times and refill with fresh water. Be sure to cook beans for at least 1 hour. Note that some people cannot tolerate certain legumes, such as garbanzos or lentils, well. If so, then these will consistently produce gas. (Bowel bacteria break down sugars called *trisaccharides* that are not well-absorbed in the small intestine.) Also, avoid allergenic foods, especially pasteurized milk products. Gas is a common symptom of lactose intolerance. Try taking a good *Lactobacillus acidophilus* supplement after eating dairy; substitute yogurt for milk.

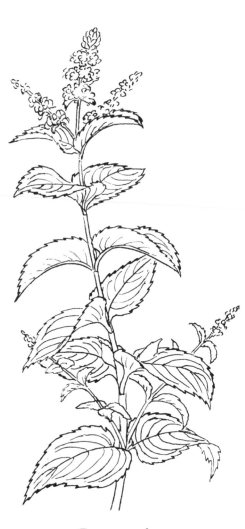

Peppermint
Mentha piperita officinalis

Herbal recommendations: Carry a small vial of peppermint oil with you at all times. Whenever you need to, place 2 or 3 drops of this oil in a cup of hot peppermint tea or hot water, stir well, and drink. Peppermint tea is also helpful, but not as strong as the oil. The following blend of traditional carminative or gas-relieving herbs is also helpful as a tea.

Other recommendations: Beneficial bacterial should be taken consistently. Take at least 10 billion organisms per day if symptoms are severe, or 3 to 6 million if less severe. Certain stretching of yoga postures can help relieve gas. Lie on the floor face-down, put your arms under your head and your rear end up in the air. Also, try massaging the abdominal area in circular, clockwise motions. Or, take an enema, one of the quickest remedies for gas known. The vacuum created as the enema water is expelled can literally suck out any gas caught in the bowels.

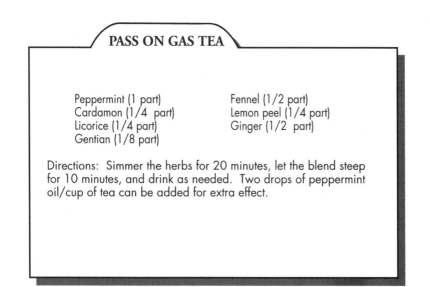

PASS ON GAS TEA

Peppermint (1 part)   Fennel (1/2 part)
Cardamon (1/4 part)   Lemon peel (1/4 part)
Licorice (1/4 part)   Ginger (1/2 part)
Gentian (1/8 part)

Directions: Simmer the herbs for 20 minutes, let the blend steep for 10 minutes, and drink as needed. Two drops of peppermint oil/cup of tea can be added for extra effect.

SKIN DISORDERS
(ACNE, PSORIASIS)

Diagnostic symptoms: Acne or psoriasis. Skin is irritated, red, oily, itchy, and inflamed. Bowel movements may have a strong, unpleasant odor.

Dietary recommendations: Although mainstream dermatologists generally do not consider diet to play a role in acne, I can assure you that it does. I suffered from acne for many years when I was younger, and I learned by trial, error, and education what did and did not work. Since then, I have used natural remedies with many people to help alleviate this problem. I have found that, as far as food goes, it is important to make 70-80% of the diet whole, natural, unprocessed foods. Focus on steamed and raw vegetables, whole grains and legumes, and fish or chicken (if desired). Strictly avoid processed foods with a high oil content, such as candy bars, chips, ice cream, and pizza. Be moderate with dairy products—eat only small amounts of cheese; use olive oil instead of butter; and avoid pasteurized cow's milk. If you do nothing else but follow this diet, I can almost guarantee results within a month or so.

Herbal recommendations: Take cool and cleansing herbs. I like dandelion, burdock root, and burdock seed as liver/skin cleansers. Oregon grape root is a classic for skin conditions in general. Milk thistle seed extract is the most remarkable herb for psoriasis. One doctor I know who has used this extract in treating psoriasis has found that at least 50% of his clients improve both clinically and subjectively. Milk thistle has been used widely in Europe, proving highly effective in protecting the liver from environmental toxins and excess free radicals (see my booklet *Milk Thistle, the Liver Herb* for more information). Milk thistle also works inside the liver cells to increase the production of proteins and enzymes, thus helping damaged tissues to rebuild themselves. It is a most amazing herb, and I highly recommend it. I also recommend the following tea as a general skin cleanser:

Other natural therapies: Apply hot and cold hydrotherapy to affected parts. First use hot compresses, or simply splash the face repeatedly with hot water, until a good flush occurs. Then repeat the process with cold water, though with about half the number of splashes. Hydrotherapy brings fresh blood to the affected skin, stimulating a general increase of deep circulation in the area. Ideally, you should repeat this procedure several times a day. However, if that is not possible, do it at least first thing in the morning and just before retiring at night.

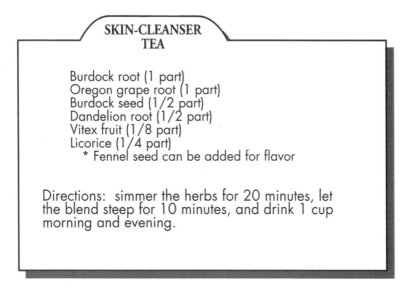

SKIN-CLEANSER TEA

Burdock root (1 part)
Oregon grape root (1 part)
Burdock seed (1/2 part)
Dandelion root (1/2 part)
Vitex fruit (1/8 part)
Licorice (1/4 part)
    * Fennel seed can be added for flavor

Directions: simmer the herbs for 20 minutes, let the blend steep for 10 minutes, and drink 1 cup morning and evening.

Hydrotherapy will also remove excess oil and dirt particles from the skin, making the use of commercial soaps unnecessary. Soap disrupts the natural protective coating of fatty acids and microflora on the skin, thus inviting pathogenic bacteria to set up camp. I have not used soap on my skin for over 15 years (except on my hands to remove grease and stubborn dirt). In that time, hydrotherapy has made my skin healthier and clearer than before. I have also seen many other cases in which these two factors—improved circulation and proper cleansing—have eliminated chronic acne.

EMOTIONAL IMBALANCES

Diagnostic symptoms: Excessive or lingering anger, sadness, or depression.

Dietary recommendations: Keep the liver open and clear by using liver flushes, walking and deep breathing, and the dietary recommendations outlined on page 22. Overeating is common in excessive emotional states, which only compounds the problem by further overloading the liver. The remedy is to eat lightly and to eat more fresh fruits and vegetables.

Herbal recommendations: I recommend the herbal tea listed below:

Other natural therapies: Try to release "stuck" emotions in constructive ways, such as heavy exercise or physical work. Crying and laughing, as long as they are not excessive, are helpful. Aromatherapy (the use of herbal scents) is also valuable in balancing emotional states. Try smelling lavender oil every so often during the day to brighten your spirits. I often carry a fresh, flowering top of lavender in my pocket to sniff whenever I feel the need. Bach flower remedies (a well known aromatherapy method) work particularly well with emotional states. I recommend seeking out a Bach flower practitioner or qualified psychologist or marriage and family counselor when dealing with long-term emotional imbalances.

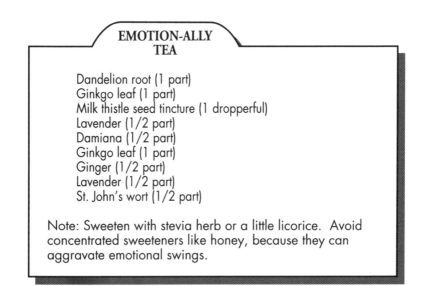

EMOTION-ALLY TEA

Dandelion root (1 part)
Ginkgo leaf (1 part)
Milk thistle seed tincture (1 dropperful)
Lavender (1/2 part)
Damiana (1/2 part)
Ginkgo leaf (1 part)
Ginger (1/2 part)
Lavender (1/2 part)
St. John's wort (1/2 part)

Note: Sweeten with stevia herb or a little licorice. Avoid concentrated sweeteners like honey, because they can aggravate emotional swings.

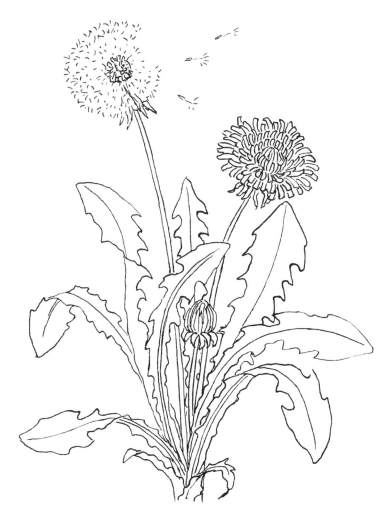

Dandelion
Taraxacum officinale

HEPATITIS OR CIRRHOSIS
(LIVER FIRE OR HEAT IN TCM)

Please note: Hepatitis and cirrhosis are serious diseases that require the attention of a qualified health practitioner or doctor.

Diagnostic symptoms: Cirrhosis is a chronic, pathological inflammation of the liver, usually resulting in scarring and loss of liver function. In extreme forms it is potentially lethal. Cirrhosis can be caused by chronic hepatitis, or alcohol and drug abuse. Signs and symptoms of hepatitis and/or cirrhosis include extreme fatigue, jaundice, headaches, facial flushing, red and inflamed gums, tenderness in liver area, diarrhea or loose, watery stools, yellow coating on tongue, near back. Hypertension and migraines are also possible. I had hepatitis twice 25 years ago, so I am very familiar with the symptoms.

Dietary recommendations: First of all, remove the stress factors that are creating the inflammation in the first place, whether they be excessive alcohol, drugs, or fried, spicy, and heavy foods (such as large quantities of red meat). Note that some cases of hepatitis are caused by an auto-immune disorder in which the body's own immune system attacks the liver. If this is the case, try a regimen of ginkgo leaf extract (24%) at 2-3 40 mg tablets per day, plus a few months of deep immune-strengthening herbs such as astragalus, ligustrum, codonopsis, shiitake, and reishi (take these as a tea or buy a commercial preparation). However, please note that it is difficult to differentiate between auto-immune and other types of hepatitis. For this reason, if the symptoms seem to worsen, or if no benefit is seen with the immune herbs, discontinue taking them. Again, with a serious disease such as hepatitis, it is always advised that you work directly with a qualified health practitioner to receive a whole program.

A light diet built on greens, grains, and legumes is the best. Don't eat too many raw foods—take them lightly steamed instead. "Superfoods" rich in micro-nutrients and high-quality proteins are essential. These include steamed nettles, spirulina or other blue-green algae, and whole almonds (if your digestion is weak, soak the nuts in water overnight). Walnuts, too, contain valuable proteins and omega-3 fatty acids that can help decrease inflammation in the body. Keep the eliminative channels open by drinking plenty of pure water. Avoid spicy, warming foods such as garlic, cayenne, hot peppers, and curries. Let food cool to almost room temperature before eating. Also, as usual, don't cook foods in fat or oil for awhile—steam them instead.

Herbal recommendations: The major herb for hepatitis and cirrhosis is milk thistle *(Silybum marianum)*. Take it as a tablet in concentrated, powdered, extract form. An average therapeutic dose of the 75% or 80% standardized extract is 1 tablet 3-4 times daily. A 10% standardized extract is also available, often blended with other liver-protective and healing herbs such as turmeric, artichoke leaf, gentian, and ginger. Of this latter preparation, take 1-2 tablets 3 times daily.

Try the following herb formula as a tea. Drink 1-3 cups per day, if it seems helpful.

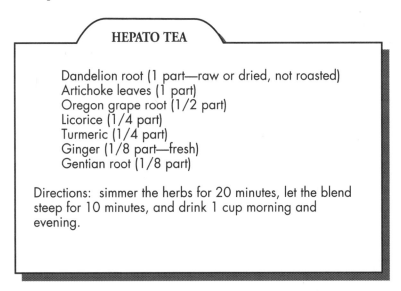

HEPATO TEA

Dandelion root (1 part—raw or dried, not roasted)
Artichoke leaves (1 part)
Oregon grape root (1/2 part)
Licorice (1/4 part)
Turmeric (1/4 part)
Ginger (1/8 part—fresh)
Gentian root (1/8 part)

Directions: simmer the herbs for 20 minutes, let the blend steep for 10 minutes, and drink 1 cup morning and evening.

Other natural therapies: Moderate walking and deep breathing are helpful. Antioxidant herbs, such as rosemary, hawthorn, and ginkgo, can be taken in addition to the above formula if the liver heat derives from heavy processing of toxins.

DRUG ADDICTIONS
(WITH ACCOMPANYING LIVER STRESS)

Diagnostic symptoms: In addiction, even after one stops using the drug, usually some of the addictive substance remains circulating in the body for a time. This perpetuates the craving for it, which makes kicking habits a challenge—as I'm sure many readers know. Both nicotine and THC (the active principle in marijuana), for instance, remain in the body long after one quits smoking. The thing to do, then, is to eliminate all traces of old drugs from the body, and this often takes a few weeks or even months of cleansing.

Dietary recommendations: The liver flush is ideal for removing drug-related toxins from the body. Add to this fasting with fresh vegetable and fruit juices as a means to quickly eliminate addictive substances. Fast for 3-5 days at a time, eating mostly steamed and raw vegetables afterwards. See the sidebar on fasting, p. 25. For extra cleansing, eat only fruits between fasts. Some sweating and lots of fresh water and oxygen (deep breathing and vigorous exercise) will also help with the process of elimination.

Note: If you are very weak, fatigued, and run-down, do not fast on juices, but use the kitcheree fast—eat several bowls of cooked soupy rice and aduki or mung beans.

Herbal recommendations: Here's my formula for eliminating addictions.

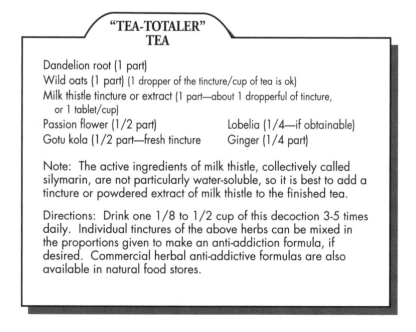

"TEA-TOTALER" TEA

Dandelion root (1 part)
Wild oats (1 part) (1 dropper of the tincture/cup of tea is ok)
Milk thistle tincture or extract (1 part—about 1 dropperful of tincture, or 1 tablet/cup)
Passion flower (1/2 part)   Lobelia (1/4—if obtainable)
Gotu kola (1/2 part—fresh tincture   Ginger (1/4 part)

Note: The active ingredients of milk thistle, collectively called silymarin, are not particularly water-soluble, so it is best to add a tincture or powdered extract of milk thistle to the finished tea.

Directions: Drink one 1/8 to 1/2 cup of this decoction 3-5 times daily. Individual tinctures of the above herbs can be mixed in the proportions given to make an anti-addiction formula, if desired. Commercial herbal anti-addictive formulas are also available in natural food stores.

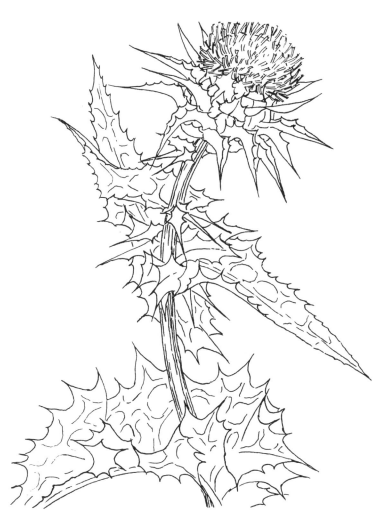

Milk Thistle
Silybum marianum

A word about golden seal: I have been asked about using this to pass drug detection tests so many times that I've lost count. Using golden seal in this manner has become something of a fad, and thousands of bottles of the herb are apparently being sold in health food stores all over the country for this purpose. However, according to the research that Steven Foster (1989) did on the subject, there is no clinical or laboratory basis for this use. My own theory on the matter is that beyond any placebo effect golden seal might have (I have had people tell me emphatically that it worked for them), the herb might have an overall cleansing effect on the liver, thus enhancing the body's eliminative process. If this is so, the tea and other recommendations in this section would certainly be more effective than pure golden seal.

Also, I must warn you that golden seal is potentially toxic if taken for more than 10-14 days in large amounts, and it is contraindicated for people with weak digestion. Do not take golden seal during pregnancy or breast-feeding.

Incidentally, if you want to kick the coffee habit, you can brew a nice cup of coffee-substitute (what we call "fake coffee") using roasted chicory and dandelion (add a kitchen spice or two, such as ginger, cardamon, or fennel, for warming action and flavor enhancement).

A basic program for fast drug elimination would include bile activators (such as yellow dock, oregon grape, and artichoke leaf), blood purifiers (such as red clover compound: red clover, burdock, dandelion, sarsaparilla), and a sauna 2-3 times in a week, using the following tea during the sweat.

Sweat Tea

Yarrow tops (1 part)

Elder flowers (1 part)

Peppermint leaf (1 part)

Make up a quart and drink 1-3 cups of the tea warm to hot.

Note: Make sure to check with your health practitioner or physician if you have heart disease or other imbalances that would be worsened by the high heat of a sauna. It is important to replace your electrolytes (potassium and other mineral salts). A good nutritional supplement with whole food and herb extracts will work fine. Or add 1 tsp of Dr. Bronners Balanced Amino Boullion to a little water and drink.

PROTECTION AGAINST ENVIRONMENTAL TOXINS

Diagnostic symptoms: Unexplained dizziness, ringing in the ears, nausea, fatigue, and "spaciness" can have a number of causes, but if they are experienced regularly, you should at least consider that sensitivity to chemical pollutants may be a factor. Toxic metals like lead and mercury are ubiquitous nowadays, having found their way into dental fillings and many other products, too. For a complete treatise on these issues, see Debra Dadd's excellent book, *Non-Toxic, Natural, and Earthwise.*

Dietary recommendations: As we've already discussed, most liver damage from environmental chemicals is thought to be due to excess free radicals. For this reason, it is good to add antioxidants and antioxidant-containing foods to the diet. I recommend vitamin E, beta-carotene, vitamin C, zinc, and selenium supplements (the latter two blended in a general nutritional supplement, not as isolated, single nutrients) during times of suspected toxic chemical stress. For regular maintenance, I suggest a program of spirulina (very high in beta-carotene), fresh greens, and liver flushes.

Herbal recommendations: The following herbal formula can be helpful. It invigorates bile flow, protects and detoxifies the liver, and stimulates phagocytosis to dispose of poisonous chemicals.

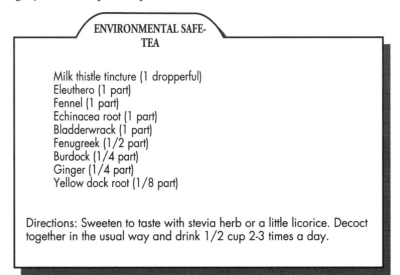

ENVIRONMENTAL SAFE-TEA

Milk thistle tincture (1 dropperful)
Eleuthero (1 part)
Fennel (1 part)
Echinacea root (1 part)
Bladderwrack (1 part)
Fenugreek (1/2 part)
Burdock (1/4 part)
Ginger (1/4 part)
Yellow dock root (1/8 part)

Directions: Sweeten to taste with stevia herb or a little licorice. Decoct together in the usual way and drink 1/2 cup 2-3 times a day.

Other natural therapies: Exercise, sweating (saunas), and intestinal cleansing are useful adjuncts. One excellent intestinal cleanser is fruit pectin powder, which has been used extensively in Russia for removing environmental toxins and radiation from the body. Take 1-3 tablespoons of the powder in water or fresh-squeezed fruit juice first thing in the morning and follow with 2 glasses of water or herb tea. Bentonite clay is another good bowel cleanser. Put 1 teaspoonful in a glass of water, stir, and leave the mixture in the sun for a few hours to ionize the clay's micro-particles. When these particles are charged, they attract and bind toxins, thus helping to pass them from the body. One enema a day is also desirable during any cleansing.

Congratulations! If you've read this far, you've learned a lot about the liver and natural liver therapy. Here's a final summary of the most important points you should remember about regaining or maintaining liver health:

9 IMPORTANT POINTS FOR OPTIMUM LIVER HEALTH

1. Lower your fat intake. Eat less refined, cooked oils and fats. Obtain essential oils from whole nuts and seeds.

2. Rest the digestive system whenever possible. Don't eat too late at night or too early in the morning. Don't eat when not hungry, and especially never overeat.

3. Be aware of proper food combining. Sweet fruit and cooked protein are the worst combination, causing fermentation.

4. Liver flushes and drinking lemon-water keep the liver moisturized and free-flowing.

5. Keep the eliminative channels open and free. Exercise to eliminate toxins via the lungs and skin. Have at least 1 bowel movement a day.

6. Massage the liver area at least once a day to help remove congestion.

7. Worry or anger can get stuck in the liver. Release these emotions in a constructive way.

8. Antioxidants such as vitamins E and C, beta-carotene, zinc, and selenium protect against toxins. Herbal antioxidants are superior to synthetic vitamins, though both can be used together.

9. Herbal formulas to cleanse, protect, and stimulate the liver are highly recommended. Teas for long-term use include: a blend of roasted dandelion, chicory, and ginger; Puri-Tea; Polari-Tea; or any of the teas discussed in pages 20-55. Milk thistle is a must for rebuilding the liver when it has been compromised or weakened in any way.

REFERENCES

GENERAL REFERENCES

American Medical Association. 1986. *Drug Evaluations*. Chicago: American Medicial Association.

Bragg, P. 1976. *The Miracle of Fasting*. Santa Barbara: Health Science.

Cheung, CS (1983). The Liver and Gall Bladder, *J Am Col Trad Ch Med* 2: 30.

Davis, B., et al. (1985). *Conceptual Human Physiology*. Columbus: Charles E. Merrill Publishing Company.

Farnsworth, NR (1980). "Botanical Sources of Fertility Regulating Agents: Chemistry and Pharmacology" in *Progress in Hormone Biochemistry and Pharmacology*, v. 1. Lancaster, England: Eden Press.

Hikino H (1986). Antihepatotoxic Actions of Allium sativum Bulbs, *Planta Medica*: 163.

Hobbs, C (1992). *Foundations of Health*. Capitola, CA: Botanica Press.

Hobbs, C (1992). *Milk Thistle: The Liver Herb*. Capitola, CA: Botanica Press.

Kaptchuk, TJ (1983). *The Web That Has no Weaver*, NY: Congdon & Weed.

Kimura Y, et al. (1984). Studies on Scutellariae Radix; IX-New Component Inhibiting Lipid Peroxidation in Rat Liver, *Planta Medica* 50: 290.

Kimura Y, et al. (1985). Effects of Extracts of Leaves of Artemisia Species....on Lipid Metabolic Injury in Rats Fed Peroxidized Oil, *Chem Pharm Bull* 33: 2028-2034.

Kiso Y, et al. (1985). Mechanism of Antihepatoxic Activity of Wuweisisu C and Gomisin A, *Planta Medica*: 331-334.

Kiso Y, et al. (1984). Antihepatotoxic Principles of Artemisia capillaris Buds, *Planta Medica*: 81.

Maeda S, et al. (1985). Effects of Gomisin A on Liver Functions in Hepatotoxic Chemicals-Treated Rats, *Japan J Pharmacol* 38: 347-353.

Maiwald, L. 1987. Bitterstoffe. *Zeitschrift fur Phytotherapie* 8: 186-88.

Raloff, J. 1993. EcoCancers. *Science News* 143: 10-13.

Reynolds, ES (1980). "Liver and Biliary Tree" in *Systemic Reactions to Injury by Environmental Agents*, p. 248.

Reynolds ES (1980). "Free-Radical Damage in Liver", *Free Radicals in Biology*, Vol. IV, p. 49.

Rose, RC, et al. (1986). Transport and Metabolism of Vitamins, *Federation Proceedings* 45: 30.

Salbe AD and Bjeldanes LF (1985). The Effects of Dietary Brussel Sprouts and Schizandra chinensis on the Xenobiotic-Metabolizing Enzymes of the Rat Small Intestines. *Food Chem Toxic* 23: 57.

Salunkhe DK, et al. (date missing). Anticancer Agents of Plant Origin, *CRC Critical Reviews in Plant Sciences*; Vol. 1, Issue 3: 218.

Tiantong B, et al. (1980). A Comparison of the Pharmacologic Actions of 7 Constituents Isolated From Fructus Schizandrae, *Chinese Med J 93*: 41-47.

Veith, I. 1972. *The Yellow Emperor's Classic of Internal Medicine*. Berkeley: University of California Press.

Vogel, A (1962). *The Liver*, Bioforce-Verlag Teufen, Switzerland.

NUMBERED REFERENCES

1. 6th Special Report to the U.S. Congress on Alcohol and Health, Jan., 1987.

2. Personal communication, May, 1987—National Clearing House on Drug Addiction.

3. U.S. Statistical Abstracts, 1984.

REFERENCES FOR WESTERN HERBALISM

Bradley, P. R. 1992. *British Herbal Compendium*, vol. 1. Dorste, England: British Herbal Medical Association.

Felter, H.W. & J.U. Lloyd. 1898. *King's American Dispensatory*. Cincinnati: The Ohio Valley Co.

Leung, A.Y. 1980. *Encyclopedia of Natural Ingredients*. New York: John Wiley & Sons.

Tierra, M. 1988. *Planetary Herbology*. Santa Fe: Lotus Press.

REFERENCES FOR TRADITIONAL CHINESE MEDICINE

Bensky, D. & A. Gamble. 1986. *Chinese Herbal Medicine, Materia Medica.* Seattle: Eastland Press.

Bensky, D. & R. Barolet. 1990. *Chinese Herbal Medicine—Formulas and Strategies.* Seattle: Eastland Press.

Chang, H.-M. & P.P.-H. But. 1986. *Pharmacology and Applications of Chinese Materia Medica*, 2 vol.'s. Philadelphia: World Scientific.

Chang, H.M., et al. 1985. *Advances in Chinese Medicinal Materials Research.* Philadelphia: World Press.

Fratkin, J. 1986. *Chinese Herbal Patent Formulas—A Practical Guide.* Santa Fe: Shya Publications.

Hsu, H.-Y. , et al. 1986. *Oriental Materia Medica, a concise guide.* Long Beach, CA: Oriental Healing Arts Institute.

Yeung, H.-C. 1985. *Handbook of Chinese Herbs and Formulas,* 2 vols. Los Angeles: Institute of Chinese Medicine.